Praise for *Skin Rules* and Debra Jaliman, M.D.

"I love this book! And so will every other woman who cares about the way she looks. Dr. Debra Jaliman has turned out a real gem, full of detailed information about the best products to use and lots of other useful tips about beauty in general. I'll never again go shopping for skin products without a Debra Jaliman list."

—Barbara Taylor Bradford,
author of *Playing the Game*

"What a remarkable book—accessible, helpful, and to the point! Every woman should have it by her bed or at her desk."   —Olympia Dukakis

"For years, glamorous New Yorkers have sought out Dr. Jaliman to look their best. This book has great, useful, and fun information!"

—Jana Klauer, M.D., author of *How the Rich Get Thin*
and *The Park Avenue Nutritionist's Plan*

"All of my famous Hollywood clients go to Debra Jaliman to maintain their youthful appearance. She is down to earth and never kisses and tells. I love *Skin Rules,* especially tip #23 regarding getting moles checked, because Debra discovered a bad mole on me that other doctors had missed."

—Susan Ciminelli, author of *The Ciminelli Solution:
A 7-Day Plan for Radiant Skin*

"I absolutely loved this very straightforward and informative guide to skin care. Dr. Jaliman provides excellent advice and tips on a wide variety of skin-care topics, from the best inexpensive products to describing the latest dermatological procedures." —Sela Ward, actress

"Debra Jaliman's clear and comprehensive book on skin care is refreshingly accessible, and as expert as we all know that she herself is. She has generously included the names of numerous, readily available products to help with the regimes she prescribes, and of course she has her own superb line of products, too. The overall message is that with proper, educated care and Debra's guidance, we can all have healthy, beautiful skin. This book is terrific." —Ali McGraw, actress

"If you care about your image, you should have Dr. Debra Jaliman on speed dial and a copy of *Skin Rules* always at hand."
—Donny Deutsch, television personality, advertising executive, and author of *Often Wrong, Never in Doubt*

"*Skin Rules*—very informative and easy to understand. This book should be required reading for all adolescents and anyone with skin problems. I was fortunate to have parents that taught me the 'cardinal' rule of clear skin. I love that one doesn't have to go to the dermatologist or buy expensive creams for every outbreak." —Katharine Ross, actress

SKIN RULES

Trade Secrets from a Top New York Dermatologist

....

DEBRA JALIMAN, M.D.

St. Martin's Griffin

New York

TO MY FAMILY,

WHO ALWAYS BELIEVED IN ME

SKIN RULES. Copyright © 2012 by Debra Jaliman, M.D. All rights reserved. Printed in the United States of America. For information, address St. Martin's Press, 175 Fifth Avenue, New York, N.Y. 10010.

www.stmartins.com

The Library of Congress has cataloged the
hardcover edition as follows:

Jaliman, Debra.
    Skin rules : trade secrets from a top New York dermatologist / Debra Jaliman. — 1st ed.
        p. cm.
    ISBN 978-1-250-00095-8 (hardcover)
    ISBN 978-1-4299-4154-9 (e-book)
    1. Skin—Care and hygiene.   2. Beauty, Personal.   I. Title.
    RL87.J35 2012
    646.7'26—dc23

                                                    2011041855

ISBN 978-1-250-02510-4 (trade paperback)

St. Martin's Griffin books may be purchased for educational, business, or promotional use. For information on bulk purchases, please contact Macmillan Corporate and Premium Sales Department at 1-800-221-7945 extension 5442 or write specialmarkets@macmillan.com.

First St. Martin's Griffin Edition: March 2013

10 9 8 7 6 5 4 3 2 1

Contents

Introduction

I have been practicing dermatology in Manhattan for more than twenty-five years as an attending physician at Mount Sinai Medical Center, where I also teach dermatology, and at my own private practice on Fifth Avenue. My patients come from all walks of life and all over the world, from the average Joe to the people you see on the cover of *Vogue* or accepting Academy Awards. Although it is certainly nice to have so many famous patients, I also take great pride when my patients bring in their sisters or best friends. Word-of-mouth referral is the highest compliment, especially when I hear "I love my skin. I can't believe how great it looks now!"

A good dermatologist—one who is well versed in the latest technology and has an artist's eye and a steady hand when it comes to fillers and Botox—can make an astounding difference in the way people look. It's not just faces that can be improved; cosmetic dermatology has expanded its benefits to the entire body. I regularly see my celebrity patients being interviewed on television. Every time I hear them ascribe their taut bodies and youthful looks to clean living and good genes, I smile to myself and think, "More like a good dermatologist."

There is so much conflicting advice in magazines, books, and Web sites that people get understandably confused and overwhelmed. I wanted to write a book that is short, practical, and to the point, one that explains not only basic skin care but also the very latest technologies that many people are unaware of. I believe that an informed person is in a better position to make the right choices. People who read this book will know what type of laser works on red skin or what radio frequency can do for the face and body. They will also know which ingredients to look for and which to avoid, depending upon their skin. My patients tell me that I have gotten them into the habit of reading the ingredient list of every skin-care product they buy. Sometimes they even save money because some excellent products are sold in drugstores. The truth is that good skin care does not have to be complicated and it does not have to be expensive, outside certain special procedures that should be done only in a board-certified dermatologist's office.

This is the decade of dermatology and its noninvasive, low-risk procedures. Many people don't know that their bellies can be tightened or their sagging eyelids lifted without cutting, all at their dermatologist's office. The proper skin care can make people look ten to fifteen years younger without resorting to plastic surgery.

Although I have worked with companies in product development in the past, I want to make it clear that I am not a paid consultant for any of the companies whose products or technologies I recommend in this book. I have my own line of skin-care products (which is excellent, by the way), but I do not mention it at all among the products I recommend because I want my recommendations to be impartial, and I really can't be expected to be impartial about the skin-care line I've developed. Every single product or technology mentioned in this book has been chosen based on my personal and professional experience and the valuable feedback I get from my patients. Since I absolutely believe that nobody has to go broke to look better, I have tried to provide less expensive alternatives whenever possible.

Few people have naturally perfect skin, but no matter what skin you were born with, it can be made to look better—usually a whole lot better. What everybody should aim for is their own best skin, the kind that gets compliments and has a healthy glow.

These seventy seven simple rules are designed to help you navigate the beauty aisles in stores and ask the right questions when you visit a dermatologist. They are the same advice I give my patients in my private practice. If you've always dreamed of having virtually flawless skin or want to look years younger than your age, this book will set you on the right track.

This paperback edition contains the latest information on new products and technologies. The skin-care industry is rapidly evolving, and beauty products are being discontinued and replaced with new ones that reflect the latest scientific advances. New body-sculpting technologies can be used to reduce fat almost anywhere on the body, and optical-imaging systems can now find melanomas of any size. It's a brave new world in dermatology practices, and patients will reap the benefits.

ONE

Don't Waste Money on

Expensive Cleansers—

Spend It on Moisturizers,

Sunscreens, and

Antiaging Products Instead

ricey skin-care lines usually include pricey cleansers, but the truth is some of the best cleansers I know are sold on drugstore shelves, so look there first. This is the advice I give to all my patients, even to the celebrities whose faces you see on magazine covers, who can certainly afford really, really expensive cleansers. "You're just washing money down the drain," I tell them. It isn't worth it to spend a lot of money on cleansers. Believe me, you can put your money to better use.

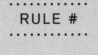

RULE #

TWO

The Right

Cleanser Is Key

One of the first questions I ask a new patient is "What do you use to cleanse your face?" The right cleanser can make a big difference; after all, it's something you use twice a day (or should). Far too often, I find that people are using the wrong cleanser. For dry, sensitive, or normal skin, buy a cleanser that is mild and won't strip the natural oils. **Neutrogena Extra Gentle Cleanser** is one of my favorites since it is fragrance-free, nondrying, and noncomedogenic (it won't clog pores). **CeraVe Hydrating Cleanser** is another good choice because it has ceramides and hyaluronic acid, which prevent skin from drying out. If you prefer a cleansing bar, **Basis Sensitive Skin Bar** or **Cetaphil** will work. Many of my patients like **Cetaphil Gentle Skin Cleanser.** I'm not crazy about its gloppy texture, but it's certainly mild enough for sensitive skin. For oily or acne-prone skin, an exfoliating cleanser will help to remove dead skin cells and bacteria. Two good options are **Derm-alogica Clean Start Wash Off Cleanser** and **L'Oreal Youth Code Foaming Gel Cleanser,** which contain salicylic acid. Although most of the salicylic acid will be washed down the drain, it does help to remove surface skin and excess oil.

THREE

Makeup Removal and

Cleansing

Are Not the Same

f you use heavy makeup, you have to remove it before cleansing. If you're wearing mascara and eye makeup, wipe that off first with an eye makeup removal product. Remember to wipe gently because the skin around the eyes is very delicate. Now for the rest of the face: Take a cotton pad and moisten it with toner or a tiny bit of water and a dab of cleanser. Make sure to remove all makeup, especially in areas where it tends to collect, such as above and in the eyebrows and in the creases around the nose and mouth.

I appear on TV fairly frequently and if there's one thing I hate, it's the heavy makeup they slather on me before I go on camera. I know it's necessary (the new high-definition technology really brings out every flaw), but I can't wait to get it off. The minute I'm off the air I run to my bag for the cotton squares and the small bottle of toner I always carry and wipe it off as fast as possible. Why toner? Because I find it's faster and more efficient than cleanser. But if you want to use cleanser, go right ahead. Once makeup is off, proceed to cleansing.

FOUR

Wash Your Face

Correctly

n my practice, we always teach patients how to cleanse their faces. The first thing they learn is that their fingers are not enough and will never get their skin really clean. Fingers can't exfoliate and besides, bacteria lurk under fingernails. So use cotton pads or rounds or a fresh washcloth every time you wash your face. Don't scrub; just rub gently, particularly around the nose and on the neck. Try it; you'll be surprised by how much cleaner your skin feels afterward. Use lukewarm water, not hot or icy cold. If you're into gadgets, one of my favorites is the **Clarisonic Sonic Skin Cleansing System,** which truly does remove more makeup, dirt, and oil than manual cleansing alone. Because it leaves skin cleaner and more exfoliated, serums and treatment products penetrate better. Just be sure to change the brush head every two or three months and choose the appropriate brush for your skin type; when in doubt, use the one for delicate skin.

People prone to breakouts should use the acne-specific brush. If the Clarisonic is not in your budget, **Olay's Professional Pro-X Advanced Cleansing System** machine can be found in many drugstores and makes an acceptable alternative. Always use a mild cleanser with any machine.

FIVE

Remove Makeup Before Going to Sleep

cannot emphasize this enough: Never go to bed without cleansing your face. If you don't, the result will be clogged pores and breakouts. If the prospect of zits isn't enough to scare you into cleansing, picture what you'll look like in the morning with last night's makeup smeared all over your face. If you're really too exhausted to wash your face with water and cleanser, at least have cleansing pads by your bed and use them to wipe makeup off. **Olay** and **Aveeno** both make good cleansing pads that can go into your evening bag, if necessary.

SIX

Cleanse Every Morning and Every Evening

n the morning, cleanse your face before you put on toner (if you need it) and then apply moisturizer or sunscreen. Even if you cleansed and removed all makeup the night before, a splash of water in the morning or standing under the shower is not enough. During the night, as you sleep, bacteria build up on your skin, along with a lot of unwanted oil. So the first step is to cleanse your face with a product suitable for your skin type, and then pat dry your face gently but thoroughly. Let me emphasize that the towel should be clean, strictly for your personal use, and changed regularly. In the evening, same thing all over again, only don't forget to apply a serum or antiaging cream afterward.

SEVEN

To Tone or Not to Tone Depends on Skin Type

ompanies that make skin-care products would like people to believe that everybody should use a toner, but nothing could be further from the truth. A surprising number of people should stay away from toners. If you have eczema or rosacea, even a salicylic acid toner is not a good idea because it can be too much for sensitive or reactive skin. People with super-dry skin shouldn't use toners, either.

Toners do have their uses, though, especially for oily, combination, normal, or acne-prone skin. If your skin is oily or prone to acne, tone twice a day (morning and night). I always tell my patients that the telltale sign is the four o'clock shiny nose; if that's what yours looks like in the afternoon, you should tone twice a day. If you have normal or combination skin, tone only once daily. If you have sensitive skin and have a hard time finding a toner you can tolerate, but you still want the benefits, here's a tip: Gently wipe some over your face and then immediately rinse it off with cool water. This also works in winter when skin is drier. A good mild toner is **Kiehl's Cucumber Herbal Alcohol-Free Toner.**

EIGHT

Exfoliate, Exfoliate, Exfoliate

Even the best skin in the world will look dull if it is not well exfoliated. You can exfoliate on a daily basis with your cotton washcloth or a disposable cotton pad and a cleanser, or with the use of the **Clarisonic** machine. If you have sensitive skin and want to use the Clarisonic, make sure to use the blue brush for delicate skin. If you have normal or oily skin, in addition to your daily exfoliation, once or twice a week use something stronger, like a scrub with fine granules or microspheres, such as **Avène Gentle Purifying Scrub.** If you don't want to use abrasive scrubs, toners and pads with alpha-hydroxy acids or salicylic acid work well, too. Just be careful not to go at your face as if you were scrubbing a frying pan. A toner or pad is meant to be wiped gently over the face once—that's it. Two toners that work well are **Vichy Laboratories Normaderm 3-in-1 Unclogging Purifying Toner** and **Clinique Mild Clarifying**

Lotion. For oily and acne-prone skin, **La Roche-Posay Effaclar Toner Astringent Lotion** is very effective. In my practice we make our own exfoliating pads, but **Trish McEvoy's Even Skin Beta Hydroxy Pads** work well, too. **Stridex Maximum Strength Pads** have 2 percent salicylic acid, which is effective on oily skin with blocked pores.

NINE

Winter, Spring, Summer, and Fall, Use a Daily Moisturizer with Sun Protection

find that as patients' skin improves, they change what they put on their faces. Patients who were used to heavy foundations start to prefer tinted moisturizers because they no longer have flaws to conceal. This is a good thing, because tinted moisturizers make people look more youthful and glowing.

For everyday use, a moisturizer—tinted or not—with an SPF of 30 is ideal. There are many excellent products available: **Stila Sheer Tinted Moisturizer SPF 30, Josie Maran Argan Tinted Moisturizer SPF 30, Aveeno Positively Radiant SPF 30, Neutrogena Healthy Defense Enhancer Tinted Moisturizer SPF 30,** and **Lancôme Bienfait Multi-vital SPF 30** are just a few. If you have oily skin, **LORAC ProtecTINT SPF 30** and **Clarins UV Plus Day Screen SPF 40** are good choices.

TEN

Skin Changes with the

Seasons and with the Years,

and Skin Care Should

Change, Too

K eep in mind that a cleansing routine that works in winter may not work so well in summer. Plus, what worked for you a couple of years ago may no longer be effective because of age or changes in hormone levels reflected in your skin. When it comes to skin care, you should be observant and adaptable. For example, you need to change your regimen when you find yourself using blotting papers throughout the day. I remember having lunch with a friend and by chance found myself staring down into her tote bag. It was a mess of crumpled facial blotting papers, a sure sign that she needed to change to an exfoliating cleanser and toner and reconsider her use of moisturizer. I sometimes tell my patients that if they absolutely feel compelled to use the same moisturizer they used in winter, in the heat of summer, they should at least refrain from putting it on their already shiny noses.

RULE #

ELEVEN

Eyes Are Special and Need

Special Products

ome people think they can use any face cream around the eyes. Wrong, wrong, wrong. The skin in the eye area is very delicate and needs specially formulated products. Use only creams and serums that specifically say they have been ophthalmologically tested, and by all means avoid eye creams with fragrances, which can irritate the skin and cause swelling. Be careful when applying creams and serums around the eyes. Pat gently onto the under-eye area and just below the brow, but never put any on the eyelid itself. Eyelid skin is so thin that the ingredients in products can actually penetrate to the eyeball beneath.

Dark under-eye circles can make even young people look old and tired. They can be treated very successfully with prescription topical creams (containing tretinoin or hydroquinone) and lasers. Over-the-counter products with retinol and caffeine can also be helpful, such as **Neocutis Lumière Bio-Restorative Eye Cream.** Vitamin K products are useless—don't waste your money.

Those little white bumps some people get under the eyes are called milia. If small, they can be dissolved with an electric needle, but large ones have to be cut out. Do not use heavy creams around the eyes, because they can make milia worse.

TWELVE

Ditch the Fake Lashes and Grow Real Ones Instead

Fake eyelashes of any sort, including lash extensions, are a terrible idea. The glue damages the delicate skin of the eyelid and pulls out eyelashes, often permanently. Dyeing your lashes is an even worse idea and is illegal in many states for good reason, since the dye can severely damage the eye and even cause blindness. Prescription **Latisse** (bimatoprost), on the other hand, is one of the few products that actually lives up to the hype. In a matter of months, lashes truly do grow fuller, longer, and darker. They grow so long, in fact, they can even irritate the cornea. To avoid this, apply Latisse only on the outer half of the upper eyelid, never on the half closest to the tear duct and never on the lower lid. It's best to apply it in the morning, when there is less risk of transferring it to the lower lid or your pillowcase. That way, you reduce the chances of side effects, which include darkening of the eyelid, redness, itchiness, and even changes in the color of the iris (although this last one is rare). A tip: Latisse works very well on bald spots in eyebrows.

One over-the-counter product appears to work almost as well as Latisse. The active ingredient in **RapidLash** is similar to the one in Latisse. Several of my patients who've used it are very happy with the result, especially because it is a less expensive alternative. A new process, called **Lashdip,** increasingly available in salons, coats the lashes and gives the appearance of wearing mascara for several weeks. It appears to be far safer than dyeing lashes.

THIRTEEN

Everybody Needs
Sunscreen, but
Moisturizers Are a
Different Story

f your skin is oily or acne prone, you may not need a moisturizer, especially in warm weather. Just use a lightweight sunscreen lotion or powder instead. Some sunscreen lotions are designed to provide a matte finish for oily or combination skin, such as **Cetaphil Derma-control Moisturizer SPF 30, Peter Thomas Roth Ultra-Lite Oil-Free Sunblock SPF 30,** and **Journée Bio-restorative Day Cream with PSP SPF 30. Colorescience Sunforgettable Mineral Powder Brush SPF 30** or **SPF 50** comes in a self-dispensing brush. You can take it everywhere and reapply it whenever you need sun protection or a matte finish. It's popular with both my female and male patients because it is so easy to carry around.

....

RULE #

....

FOURTEEN

It's the Sun That

Ruins Skin, Not Age

People think that crinkly skin, liver spots, and wrinkles are all part of normal aging. They're not—they're just signs of sun damage. I'll never forget the patient who came in with her elderly mother. My patient had the alligator skin that comes from baking on too many beaches, and she required many expensive treatments to repair it. Her mother, on the other hand, was a Southern belle who at the age of eighty-four still had porcelain skin with remarkably few wrinkles. Her secret? She had avoided the sun all her life, she had used sunscreen and big, beautiful hats to protect her face, and, as she told me, "I've always walked on the shady side of the street." We'd all do well to copy her example.

The American Academy of Dermatology now calls for a minimum SPF (sun protection factor) of 30, so for daily use a sunscreen with SPF 30 is fine. Remember, sun damage is cumulative; even ten minutes of exposure a day over the course of a lifetime is enough to cause major problems.

FIFTEEN

Vitamin D Is Good,

but Not When It Comes

from the Sun

spend a lot of time in my practice debunking the "sunlight is good for you" myth. I can't begin to count how many patients have told me that they've heard on television that to get vitamin D they absolutely have to go out every day without sunscreen and catch some rays, even if only for ten minutes. What makes it worse is that some of these patients have already had skin cancers removed from their faces.

Let me be absolutely clear: Everybody needs vitamin D and it would be very hard to get enough of it from food alone. But the best way to get an adequate amount of vitamin D is not through damaging your skin, but through a much cheaper, easier, and effective daily supplement. I recommend that adults take at least 1,000 milligrams a day. This is especially important for people with dark skin, but even the blondest, most fair-skinned person needs a vitamin D supplement.

SIXTEEN

Choose Sunscreens
Carefully and Learn
Which Ingredients Are
Right for You

S unscreens come in two general types, chemical and physical. Chemical sunscreens are effective, but some people are allergic to the main ingredients. If you do opt for a chemical sunscreen, look for one that contains avobenzone (Parsol 1789) or Mexoryl. In Europe, Tinosorb is a widely used ingredient that seems to do an excellent job, but it has yet to be approved for use in the United States. One that is available here and that my patients like is **Anthelios SPF 40 Lotion** by **La Roche-Posay,** whose active ingredient is Mexoryl SX.

I prefer physical sunscreens that contain zinc oxide and titanium dioxide. They block more of the spectrum and have less potential to cause an allergic reaction. For people with rosacea or sensitive skin, physical sunscreens have an added benefit: Zinc oxide soothes irritation (that's why it's used on babies with diaper rash) and reduces redness. Same thing goes for people with eczema. There are many excellent physical sunscreens on the market, and most moisturizers now have a good degree of sun protection. One of my favorites is **Vanicream Sensitive Skin SPF 30,** which is gentle enough to use on babies, although adults may find it a little oily. For acne-prone skin, **Neutrogena Pure & Free Baby Faces Ultra Gentle Sunblock SPF 50+, Elta MD UV Clear SPF 46,** or **Neova Z-Silc SPF 30** are very good alternatives.

Remember, look for a moisturizer with an SPF of at least 30, even if you're going to be sitting in an office or a classroom. Keep in mind that UVA rays penetrate glass, so your skin can be damaged even when you're sitting near a window or driving a car.

SEVENTEEN

Buy Physical Sunscreens

That Are White,

Not Clear

S ome of my patients complain that sunscreens containing zinc oxide and titanium dioxide require a lot of rubbing to prevent a whitish cast. As it turns out, though, this is the property that makes these products safe to use: They appear white because the particles of zinc oxide and titanium dioxide are too big for the skin to absorb.

In sunscreens, particle size matters, not just for sun protection but for your overall health as well. This is one area where big is truly better. When sunscreens go on white, it means that they contain micronized zinc oxide or titanium dioxide. When they come out clear from the tube, the manufacturer has used nanoparticles that are many times smaller. And scientists are growing increasingly concerned about nanoparticles and their possible effects. Recent studies have shown that people whose sunscreens contain zinc nanoparticles have increased levels of zinc in their blood. This is not the case for micronized particles, which, as far as research shows, seem to be too big to penetrate the surface of the skin; in other words, they just sit there and physically block the sun's rays. Some countries now force manufacturers to disclose the use of nanoparticles on sunscreen labels, but the United States is not yet one of them.

EIGHTEEN

Toss That Old Sunscreen and Get a New One

t has been my experience that sunscreens lose potency over time and even more quickly if they are left in bright sunlight. This is especially true of chemical sunscreens that contain avobenzone (Parsol 1789). So don't leave your sunscreen out on the sand; put it back in your bag. As a rule, don't keep sunscreens from one year to another. I've treated patients who got terrible, blistering sunburns because they used an old sunscreen they found at the bottom of their beach bags.

NINETEEN

Steer Clear of Sunscreens with Retinyl Palmitate

One ingredient that should not be in sunscreen (but frequently is) is retinyl palmitate, a vitamin A derivative that is closely related to retinol. Like retinol, retinyl palmitate is safe and effective in night creams—no surprise there, since retinyl palmitate is converted to retinol on your skin. The problem lies in retinol's ability to increase cell turnover, which is exactly what you want at night. But you don't want this during the day, because those new skin cells are very sensitive and easily damaged.

I've had patients come in saying that they refuse to use sunscreen because they've read it can cause cancer. This is a very important issue, and one I want to clarify. The problem is not in sunscreen itself, but in retinyl palmitate, which breaks down in sunlight to form free radicals that can indeed harm cells and possibly lead to cancer.

But this is no reason not to use sunscreens, which are absolutely vital to protect your skin. All you have to do is buy one of the many good sunscreens that do not list retinyl palmitate among their ingredients.

TWENTY

A City Sunblock Is Not Enough for Outdoor Sports

Athletic people may be in better shape than the rest of us, but they also tend to have more sun damage if they haven't taken appropriate precautions. For sports, the beach, and the mountains, look for sunscreens with a high SPF. I recommend **L'Oreal Sublime Sun Advanced Sunscreen Crystal Clear Mist SPF 50+, Mustela High Protection Sun Lotion SPF 50,** and **Vanicream SPF 30.** The Food and Drug Administration (FDA) now specifies an SPF of no higher than 50. While lotions and creams are best for the face, I find that a spray sunscreen is easier to apply on the body, especially on the hair parting and back. A good spray is **Hampton Sun SPF 35 Continuous Mist Sunscreen.** If you want to be extra-cautious and lessen the risk of inhaling chemicals, look for a spray sunscreen in a pump bottle, not in an aerosol can. Remember, even if the sunscreen is water-resistant, you will still need to reapply it every time you come out of the water.

In the mountains, particularly on ski slopes, sunscreen is essential. **Avène High Protection Tinted Compact SPF 50** is easy to carry with you and reapply during the day. **Physicians Formula Mineral Wear Talc-Free Airbrushing Pressed Powder SPF 30** is sold in many drugstores and is a less expensive alternative.

Don't forget the tips of your ears, the back of your neck, and where your hair parts, because these areas are vulnerable to skin cancer. If you don't want to spray sunscreen on your hair or scalp, wear a hat instead. Sun-protective hats and clothing are readily available in stores and online.

TWENTY-ONE

Lips, Eyes, and Hands Need Sun Protection, Too

D ermatology isn't just about appearance; it's also about saving lives. Thousands of new cases of skin cancer on the lip are diagnosed every year; ninety percent of these are squamous cell carcinomas that can metastasize, spreading to other areas of the body. Wear a lip balm or lipstick with as high an SPF number as you can find. Opaque lipsticks with zinc oxide or titanium dioxide have some degree of protection because they act as a physical sunblock, so wearing bright red lipstick with your bathing suit is not a bad idea. Translucent lip glosses offer far less protection, but there are a few with an SPF of 30 or higher. **Colorescience Sunforgettable Lip Shine SPF 35** is a good choice. For the delicate area around the eyes, where you should not use a chemical sunscreen (unless you want your eyes to burn and sting), I like **Shiseido Eye Protection Sun Cream SPF 32.** Always wear sunglasses that provide 100 percent

UV protection, sometimes labeled as UV400; to minimize eye wrinkles from sun damage, wear wraparound glasses. And don't forget to put sunscreen on your hands! Hands can give away your age in an instant. You don't want to spend time and money keeping up your face only to have your hands look decades older. Fortunately, hand creams now come with sun protection. For example, **Paula's Choice Resist Ultimate Anti-Aging Hand Cream SPF 30+** moisturizes and protects at the same time. **Kiehl's Crème de Corps Light Weight SPF 30 Body Lotion** and **Clarins Sunscreen Care Cream SPF 30** also work well on hands.

TWENTY-TWO

There's a Pill for That

One of the most promising advances in sun protection is **Heliocare,** an over-the-counter sunscreen pill, which has been approved by the FDA for added sun protection. It in no way replaces sunscreen or protective clothing, and it does not reverse sun damage. What it can do is provide an additional layer of protection for people with sun intolerance. The pill starts to work thirty minutes after taking the dose, so plan accordingly. If you are taking medication that makes you sensitive to the sun or if you are traveling to a very sunny place, Heliocare is worth looking into. It is now available at most drugstores.

TWENTY-THREE

That Suspicious-Looking
Mole Should Be Checked
by a Dermatologist—
So Should the Ones That
Don't Look Suspicious

t takes a trained eye to pass a verdict on moles. This can be a matter of life or death, so go straight to a dermatologist. Even a few months' delay can make a difference. A pinpoint dot that most would dismiss may be diagnosed as skin cancer. If it has to be removed, think how much smaller the scar will be if the cancer is caught early—it's just common sense. This is why a yearly body check is a good idea. I know the thought of standing naked in front of a dermatologist makes many people squirm, but the reality is nowhere near as bad as they think. In my practice, we do everything to make the experience as quick and comfortable as possible, and so will any good dermatologist. **Melafind** uses optic imaging and a hand scanner to find even tiny melanomas. It's a quick and painless procedure.

Remember: Dark skin and a family history free of skin cancer are no guarantee, so get checked.

TWENTY-FOUR

Tanning Beds and Salons Should Be Made Illegal

Y ou think that sounds harsh? Then you should hear what I tell my patients. This is the gist of it: If you want to look years older than your true age, have deep wrinkles in places you never expected, and ruin the texture and the color of your skin, a tanning salon is the place for you. Using tanning beds increases your chance of melanoma by a whopping 75 percent, particularly if you are under thirty-five. I've seen patients in their twenties who have the crow's feet of a fifty-year-old, thanks to their tanning salons. Stay away from these places. Period.

TWENTY-FIVE

For That Real, Tanned Look, Fake It

Twenty years ago, when the first self-tanners made people look like giant pumpkins, it was understandable that people preferred to get tanned by the sun. But nowadays self-tanners are so good there's no excuse for permanently damaging your skin. I once scolded a patient for her deep, bronze tan, only to find out she had used a self-tanner so good (and so expertly applied), it had fooled even me.

It takes a few hours before you see the darkening effect, which can make it tricky to get the right shade. Pick a shade that corresponds to what your skin would look like with a light tan. Don't go for a dramatically different look, because it will always look unnatural. Since we are constantly shedding the top layer of our skin cells, you will need to repeat the application once a week to maintain the color. Two of my favorite self-tanning products are **St. Tropez Bronzing Mousse** and **Clarins Self Tanning**

Instant Gel. You can also use products that gradually build up color through daily application, such as **Jergens Natural Glow Daily Moisturizer** and **L'Oréal Sublime Glow Daily Moisturizer.** I find that sprays tend to go on unevenly, so I recommend creams, mousses, gels, and lotions. Before applying a self-tanner, exfoliate in the shower with a washcloth or a nylon mesh sponge. To avoid the dreaded orange palms, use disposable gloves or wash your hands immediately after using the product. If you need to remove color from hands, the most effective remedy is **Roux Clean Touch Haircolor Stain Remover.** A word of caution about spray-on tans: Mists and sprays can be inhaled. An occasional sprayed-on tan probably does not pose a serious risk, but I would be leery of getting them routinely. Salon employees who are exposed to the sprays several times a week should take precautions.

TWENTY-SIX

It Is Definitely Possible to Have Too Much of a Good Thing

ny ingredient that is designed to change the appearance of your skin, like tretinoin, retinol, or alpha-hydroxy acids, can cause a reaction, especially if you use too much. By too much, I mean any amount larger than a pea, because that should be enough for your face. Remember, these products are designed to be used sparingly, so apply them with a light hand. I see many new patients who come in with red, peeling faces or swollen eyes because they've used these products too enthusiastically or too close to the eyes. Be very careful to stretch your skin slightly when you're applying treatment creams and lotions around the nostrils, because that's where they tend to accumulate, and when they do, they can burn the skin. You should avoid the corners of your mouth for the same reason.

TWENTY-SEVEN

Take It Nice and Slow

always tell my patients to approach skin treatment the way they approach exercise. Nobody should run a marathon the first day out on the track; by the same token, you should gradually build up a tolerance to any skin treatment. Use only one new product at a time until you are sure you are not reacting to it; then introduce another. That way, if you do react, you know the culprit. A week should be long enough.

RULE #

TWENTY-EIGHT

Proceed with Caution When It Comes to Sensitive Skin

have tremendous empathy for my patients with eczema and sensitive skin because I know exactly what it's like (which is not a bad thing for a doctor). It's only a slight exaggeration to say that throughout my childhood my face looked like a strawberry—red and perpetually covered with blotches and hives. I was allergic to just about everything. As a teenager, I could never join my friends in experimenting with makeup; if I did, my lips and eyes would swell so dramatically I would be unrecognizable. I've never grown out of it, and my skin is still highly reactive. I have to rush past the fragrance section of department stores. Theaters and planes can be problematic, and I've even had to change seats because the person next to me was doused in perfume. In short, I am living proof that skin can react to what is in the air, not just what is applied to it.

It is hard to recommend products because sensitive or

allergic people vary so greatly in their reactions. Here are a few products that I recommend for my highly sensitive patients: **Aquaphor Healing Ointment** is effective on dry, chapped, or irritated skin; **Mustela,** a European line made for babies without fragrances, colorants, preservatives, or parabens, has gentle products, from sunscreens to body washes, that are good for people with eczema; **Oilatum** unscented cleansing bars work well, too. As for the all-essential sunscreen, **Vanicream Sunscreen SPF 30** and **EltaMD UV Physical SPF 41** are the best I've found. But again, I have to say that even though these are the gentlest products I can think of, it is still possible that some people may react. The depressing truth is that people with sensitive skin can react to anything.

....

RULE #

....

TWENTY-NINE

The Washing Machine

Can Be an Unsuspected

Source of Misery

People with sensitive, itchy skin should use allergen-free detergents, such as **All Free and Clear** and **Charlie's Soap.** Avoid all softeners and dryer sheets. A tip for people with allergies and eczema: Put laundry through the rinse cycle twice to get rid of every trace of detergent.

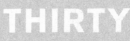

RULE #

THIRTY

Hypoallergenic Doesn't
Always Equal Safe

Anybody who has sensitive skin knows how hard it is to find the right products. Reading labels can tell you only so much, but it's unavoidable. "Hypoallergenic" is a vague and somewhat meaningless term; it just means while the chance of a reaction is reduced, it is still there. A pet peeve of mine (and that is putting it mildly) is how hard it is to find products that are truly fragrance-free. Be aware that products labeled "unscented" can still contain masking fragrances. Essential oils can also be highly irritating.

Because reactions are so individual, you may have to find the best products for your skin through trial and error. A dermatologist or an allergist can help determine your allergies. If you know what ingredients you are allergic to, you know what to avoid.

THIRTY-ONE

Take Care of Dry Skin Now So You Don't Pay Later

f you suffer from very dry skin or eczema, your ancestors may be to blame. Severely dry skin is actually hereditary and runs in families. Very dry skin should not be taken lightly because not only can it make your life uncomfortable, it also increases the risk of skin infections. Insufficient oil in the skin means that you have far less barrier protection against bacteria and viruses. Besides, dry skin itches (sometimes unbearably) and constant scratching can permanently damage skin. The best treatment consists of prescription moisturizers such as **Hylatopic Plus**, **EpiCeram**, **Mimyx**, and **Atopiclair**, which mimic the skin's natural barrier protection. An excellent over-the-counter alternative is **Vaseline Intensive Rescue Repairing Moisture Fragrance Free Lotion.**

There are other causes for dry skin, and one is spending too much time in the shower or the bathtub. I'm all for cleanliness, but try not to take more than one or two quick showers a day. Long baths in very hot water aren't a good idea, either. And some soaps and body washes, particularly those with very strong fragrances, are extremely drying. Look for mild and moisturizing body wash or bar soap, such as **Eucerin Calming Body Wash, Kiss My Face Pure Olive Oil Soap,** or **Cetaphil Gentle Cleansing Bar.** Deodorant soaps are bad, period. Use regular deodorant after your shower instead.

In over-the-counter moisturizers or lotions, look for these ingredients: humectants, such as hyaluronic acid and glycerin; lipids, such as ceramides; and emollients, such as lanolin and propylene glycol. If you are allergic to wool you should not use any product that contains lanolin; some people find that propylene glycol makes their skin itch or burn. Occlusive moisturizers (petrolatum, mineral oil, or beeswax, for example) work by forming a protective film that prevents moisture loss and assists with hydration, but they can be heavy and greasy. **Aquaphor,** for example, is inexpensive and very effective, but because it is so heavy many people prefer to use it at night.

THIRTY-TWO

Moisture Is Essential for Your Skin

Moisturize your body and face while your skin is still damp from the bath and shower, even if you use prescription creams. Remember that during the winter months indoor air can become very dry. A humidifier in your bedroom can make a big difference because by increasing water in the air it hydrates the skin. Don't forget to clean it every two weeks with a solution of equal parts of white vinegar and water. The low-tech alternative of a pot of water on the radiator works just fine, too.

THIRTY-THREE

Legs and Feet Need Extra Care

Not that this is good news, but it is perfectly possible to have a very oily face and lizard legs. The concentration of oil glands in your skin decreases as you go down the body. Almost everyone requires some moisturizing from the knees down, but some people require heavy-duty stuff, especially on the feet.

I've had patients come in with heels so dry and cracked that they bled and made it painful to walk. The first thing I always check for is fungal infections, because athlete's foot can cause very dry, rough feet. If there is no infection, I recommend a two-pronged approach. First, use a pumice stone or a foot file to get rid of the dead skin. Remember that while both are effective, they are used differently: the pumice stone on wet skin and the file on dry. My favorite file is the **Diamancel Genuine Diamond Foot Buffer,** but many of my patients like the much cheaper **Ped Egg,** which also works very well. The

Emjoi MicroPedi Foot Buffer is more expensive, but highly effective. Once feet are smooth, apply a thick layer of a very rich emollient, such as **Dr. Scholl's For Her Foot Butter, L'Occitane Shea Butter Foot Cream,** or **Badger Balm Foot Balm,** and put on white cotton socks. Do this at bedtime, and your feet will be much softer in the morning. A word of caution: Diabetics should not use a foot file or a pumice stone. A cream with glycolic or lactic acid is safer. An excellent, relatively inexpensive over-the-counter alternative to a prescription cream is **AmLactin Foot Cream,** which is sold in most drugstores.

Two groups of people are particularly susceptible to dry, cracked heels. One is menopausal women, because lower estrogen levels mean drier skin in general. The other is people with low thyroid levels. I've actually diagnosed hypothyroidism in some of my patients observing their heels and referred them to an endocrinologist for treatment.

THIRTY-FOUR

The Department Store
Is Not a Reliable Source
of Medical Advice

For that, you have to go to a dermatologist. Do not—repeat, do not—ask the people selling cosmetics for skin-care advice. I can't tell you how many times I've gone to purchase a lipstick and had a salesperson try to sell me a moisturizer for dry skin, even though my skin is so oily I should join an oil cartel. Even worse is when salespeople continue the torrent of misinformation after I tell them I am a dermatologist. The people behind the counter are there to provide help with makeup colors and make commissions on sales. Keep that in mind.

THIRTY-FIVE

Beware of Bacteria and Steer Clear of Testers

Wash your makeup brushes and sponges at least once a week. Baby shampoo is fine; just make sure to get it all out and let brushes and sponges air-dry completely. The dishwasher is fine for sponges, but it may ruin brushes. If you love your expensive brushes, the **Brush Guard Cleaning Kit** is a nifty idea.

I've seen a surprising number of patients whose acne failed to improve until they actually started washing their applicators. Keep in mind that bacteria build up quickly on any surface, particularly one that comes into contact with your skin. This is especially important to remember with eye applicators. And never, *never* use another person's mascara, or even worse, store testers that others have used. Disposable testers are no guarantee, either, because you don't know if the previous customer double dipped. At the cosmetics counter, test makeup on your wrist and arm. Don't even think of using that tester lipstick on your mouth. Better to throw out a new lipstick that turned out to be the wrong shade than to risk a herpes infection on your face. I have seen patients with herpes on lips and eyelids they got from testers, and it is not a pretty sight. Although herpes is treatable, it is a recurrent infection—one you will have to live with for the rest of your life.

THIRTY-SIX

The Best Place to Keep Your Makeup and Skin-Care Products Is in the Refrigerator

have to come clean here. I know that the warm, steamy environment of the bathroom makes products deteriorate faster, but most of the time I am as guilty as everybody else. Let's be realistic: Makeup application and skin cleansing are done in the bathroom, so that's where I and most people I know store skin-care products. Still, if you have very expensive creams or have bought several jars or lipsticks that you don't use every day, keep them in the fridge, right by the eggs and orange juice.

THIRTY-SEVEN

Use a Machine
to Polish Your Face

Home microdermabrasion systems won't give you the same results you'd get in a doctor's office, but they can certainly make your skin look better and are a good way to maintain a medical microdermabrasion between treatments. One of the best is the **DDF Revolve 400x Micro-Polishing System,** which uses sodium bicarbonate (yes, good old baking soda) crystals. It also has a brush that can be used for everyday cleansing, just like the **Clarisonic.** Warning: Don't use these machines if you have sensitive skin, rosacea, or eczema.

THIRTY-EIGHT

Go for the Glow—If Exfoliating
at Home Isn't Enough,
Have Your Skin Polished at the
Doctor's Office

Microdermabrasion really improves skin texture, eliminates superficial discoloration, and even erases very fine lines. It can leave skin glowing and looking younger in just one visit. It's very popular with my patients because it takes just twenty minutes and can literally be done during their lunch hour. However, I don't like to use microdermabrasion on people with eczema or rosacea because it can aggravate already red skin. While safe and effective when done in a dermatologist's office, this procedure can be risky when done in salons. I remember the patient who came in complaining that her eyes had been sore ever since she'd had her skin polished at a salon. Turns out that she had corneal abrasions because she hadn't been given adequate eye protection.

For years, microdermabrasion entailed using a high-pressure stream of aluminum oxide or sodium bicarbonate crystals, but the latest technology uses a diamond-tipped wand instead. The wand's great advantage is that it can be used safely around the mouth and eyes, which is where people show age the most.

Because the top layer of the skin is removed, some people's skin will turn pink for a few hours—something to take into consideration if you have to return to the office or have a big evening planned. Do not use any treatment creams, such as those with retinol, on newly polished skin for at least two days, and protect this newly revealed skin from the sun at all costs. By the way, many patients have microdermabrasion done on their chests and hands because what is the use of having a youthful, glowing face if your hands and cleavage don't match?

THIRTY-NINE

Acne Doesn't Just Ruin

Skin; It Can Ruin

Self-Esteem, Too—

Just Ask Any Teenager

see them all the time—the shy teenagers who cover their faces with their hair and stare at the floor. When I get them to look at me, I understand why, and my heart goes out to them. Acne can truly make adolescence a misery, transforming boys and girls into withdrawn, unsociable kids with painful inferiority complexes. Boys suffer just as much as girls, if not more, because daily shaving can exacerbate acne and boys don't usually wear makeup to cover it up.

If your child has acne, take action immediately. Acne treatment is covered by most insurance plans, and even if it isn't, acne is one skin condition where trying to save money can cause long-term damage. The earlier treatment is started, the less the chance of physical and emotional scars. And sometimes just one or two office visits are all that's needed to get on the right track.

Teenage acne tends to run in families, unfortunately,

and raging hormones make matters worse. Sweaty football helmets, germy cell phones, and hands perpetually cradling cheeks and chins can lead to breakouts, too. Then there are serious hormonal imbalances, such as polycystic ovarian syndrome (PCOS); I always ask teenage girls about their periods, because controlling them with appropriate birth control pills can make a big difference in their skin.

The first step to control teenage acne is proper cleansing, which should always be gentle; if the skin is very oily, an exfoliating cleanser can help. The next step is a topical treatment: antibiotics, benzoyl peroxide, retinoids, salicylic acid, glycolic acid, and maybe an anti-inflammatory such as dapsone. Cysts can be treated with steroid injections, which bring down the swelling in a day or so. For severe acne, oral medication may be necessary, such as antibiotics and for girls, hormone blockers (spironalactone). Accutane (isotretinoin) is controversial, but in cases of severe, scarring acne that has not responded to treatment, it can be a huge help.

FORTY

A Good Facial Can Unclog Pores

S ome people seem to develop blackheads and white-heads no matter what they do. When performed by a dermatologist or a trained esthetician, facials can absolutely make skin look better and help reduce acne breakouts. As long as you don't have rosacea, the steam used in facials shouldn't pose a problem. Make sure that pores are cleaned with a stainless steel comedone extractor, which exerts even pressure around the pore, and never with the fingers. Warning: Do not use any heavy creams right after a facial: they will just clog up pores again.

FORTY-ONE

Treat Red Pimples with Blue Light

A very cool technological innovation that both my teenage and adult acne patients love is blue light therapy, which destroys bacteria on the surface of the skin. Combined with a skin-care regimen and administered twice a week for four weeks, it can give impressive results. Some patients may need maintenance treatments, but people tend to be very happy with the results.

FORTY-TWO

Don't Despair If You're Over Thirty and Breaking Out— Nobody Needs to Know

hear this every week. A new patient comes in and says, "I have wrinkles and I'm still breaking out. When will this ever end?" The sad truth is that some people have acne all their adult lives, even into their eighties. But don't lose hope if you're one of them—only your dermatologist has to know.

In more than twenty-five years of practice, I haven't met a case of acne I couldn't beat—including my own. When I tell my patients that I, too, have adult acne, they roll their eyes, since my face shows no trace. But that is thanks to the skin care regimen I follow religiously—because that is what it takes to keep adult acne at bay.

Proper cleansing is essential, of course, preferably with a mild product, followed by exfoliation. I really like exfoliating pads with both glycolic and salicylic acids, because they unclog pores and make skin look more radiant. Any regimen for adult skin has to be tailored to the individual, but just as an example, here's mine. In the morning, I use a mild cleanser, followed by a quick wipe with an exfoliating pad. Then I apply a brightening lotion to even out my skin tone, followed by a sunscreen. At night, I cleanse my face and dry it carefully before applying a retinol product (retinol on wet or damp skin can be very irritating). I finish with either a light moisturizing cream or a serum.

FORTY-THREE

For the Occasional Blemish, the Drugstore Is Enough

Not everybody needs to rush to the dermatologist to get a pimple treated. If you get an occasional zit or have very mild premenstrual breakouts, you can certainly handle it on your own with the help of your local drugstore. Look for products that contain 2.5 percent benzoyl peroxide (higher concentrations are too drying) or 2 percent salicylic acid. They work differently: Benzoyl peroxide kills the bacteria that cause pimples, while salicylic acid cleans out pores. For spot treatment, two good alternatives are **Clinique Acne Solutions Spot Healing** and **Clean & Clear Advantage Acne Spot Treatment.** If you have hormonal acne and you know that you tend to break out in certain areas, say your chin, don't wait for a breakout to happen. Use salicylic acid or benzoyl peroxide on that area every day to prevent new pimples from forming. Depending on how sensitive your skin is, you can treat it every day or alternate between benzoyl peroxide one day and salicylic acid the next. It's best to use salicylic acid at night because it makes the skin more sensitive to the sun. Warning: Do not use any skin product with salicylic acid while pregnant.

If you're fond of your pretty colored sheets, be aware that benzoyl peroxide can bleach them, which is why I tell my patients to invest in white pillowcases. For people out of their teenage years, **Neutrogena Healthy Skin Anti-Blemish Anti-Wrinkle Cream,** which contains both salicylic acid and retinol, is an excellent product because it treats acne and wrinkles at the same time.

FORTY-FOUR

The Wrong Makeup Can Make Acne Worse

People with acne cannot use heavy foundations and oily concealers, period. I've had several celebrity clients whose acne did not clear up until I personally spoke to their makeup artists—all that heavy TV makeup was ruining my carefully prescribed skin-care regimen.

Every major makeup company now makes oil-free and noncomedogenic foundations. People with very oily skin can use mineral foundations, which keep skin matte longer.

FORTY-FIVE

Treatment Will Improve Acne Scars, but Don't Expect Miracles

A dermatologist can do a lot to minimize old acne scars, but chances are they won't go away completely and you will never get airbrushed skin perfection. That said, laser treatments such as the **Fraxel,** sometimes coupled with **Thermage CPT** radio frequency, can improve appearance greatly. Warning: People with darker complexions should never have ablative laser treatment, which removes the skin's top layer, because the odds are good they will end up with mottled skin; a good alternative for them is a combination of **MedLite C** laser treatments and light microdermabrasion. Deep, ice-pick scars are the hardest to treat. Hyaluronic acid injections can fill shallow scars for about a year, but sooner or later another injection will be needed. For deeper scars, I've had some success with punch skin grafts to fill them in and injections of **Sculptra** to stimulate collagen production, but they rarely disappear completely.

FORTY-SIX

Not Every Adult with Pimples Has Acne—It May Be Rosacea, Instead

Rosacea sometimes looks like acne; one way to tell them apart is that blackheads are not seen with rosacea. For extremely mild cases, try what is available in stores first: **Clinique Redness Solutions, Eucerin Redness Relief,** and **La Roche-Posay Rosaliac Anti-Redness** products are fairly easy to find. But most rosacea cases require the care of a dermatologist, and it may take several months to bring the redness under control. Topical and oral medications, such as antibiotics, can be very effective. I've started using **Pyratine XR,** a plant-based growth factor, and specially formulated green tea gels with excellent results; those are nonprescription, but usually found only in a dermatologist's office. Then there are lasers and light therapy, which can be phenomenally successful. Infrared light therapy calms inflammation, while the same blue light used on acne patients helps with rosacea breakouts. The **CoolGlide** laser seals broken vessels on the nose and cheeks. Patients who cannot go out in cold weather without their noses turning bright red love the **Genesis** laser. It may take several treatments spaced over months, but it banishes background redness and red noses.

FORTY-SEVEN

Change Diet and Habits to Get Rid of the Red

Heat, steam, and sunlight are universal triggers for rosacea, but alcohol, spicy foods, very hot beverages, heavy consumption of caffeine, MSG, and Nutrasweet (aspartame) and even fragrances can also aggravate it. Food allergies can be hard to pinpoint, so a food diary and an elimination diet are useful. Remember, zinc oxide sunscreens are essential for rosacea patients and should be used daily.

FORTY-EIGHT

Zap Away Those Broken Blood Vessels

We're not talking varicose veins here, which require a different procedure, but the faint red lines that are often seen around the nose or on the cheeks. You can conceal them with makeup for the rest of your life, but it is almost as easy to get rid of them permanently with one or two laser treatments. It's safe, it's effective, and it takes just a few minutes.

FORTY-NINE

Don't Wait Until Wrinkles Appear to Start Using Antiaging Products

Collagen production starts decreasing in the late twenties, so that's when people should start using retinols, antioxidants, and collagen boosters, especially around the eyes.

FIFTY

Antiaging Creams and Serums Aren't Just Hype

Creams and serums can do wonderful things for aging skin. In just a couple of months, skin can look markedly younger and smoother. What ages appearance is not so much wrinkles and creases, but uneven skin discoloration. A brighter, even-toned complexion can make people look ten years younger. Another benefit of antiaging products is that fine lines are noticeably decreased, even the telltale crow's feet around the eyes. In my practice, we constantly test and reformulate very effective antiaging products for our patients. However, there are also many excellent products available in stores. Look for products with DNA-repair ingredients or that contain growth factors, peptides (to stimulate collagen production), retinol, cytokinins, resveratrol, caffeine, niacin and its derivatives, vitamin C (ascorbic acid), and green tea. I've tested these drugstore and department store products and found them to be effective: **RoC Retinol Correxion**

Deep Wrinkle Serum, L'Oréal RevitaLift Anti-Wrinkle Concentrate, Skinceuticals Retinol Refining Night Cream, Philosophy Miracle Worker Pads, ZO Skin Health Ossential Growth Factor Serum, SkinMedica TNS, Boots Number 7 Protects Perfect Intense Beauty Serum, Ole Henriksen Truth Serum, Neova DNA Total Repair, Peter Thomas Roth Unwrinkle Night Cream, and Neutrogena Rapid Wrinkle Repair Serum.

FIFTY-ONE

Good Things Come in

Tubes and Pumps

For the most part, try to buy products that come in tubes or pumps because contents deteriorate quickly when exposed to air and sunlight, which happens every time a jar is opened. Now, there are some very good products that are sold only in jars; for these, you should use a cotton swab rather than your fingers. Remember, every time you stick your fingers into a jar, you are introducing bacteria into it.

FIFTY-TWO

For Instant Rejuvenation,

Get Fillers

n a matter of minutes, fillers can erase ten years, make lips more sensual, and sculpt cheekbones. I've injected fillers into actors' faces on movie sets without interrupting the day's filming schedule.

Light fillers (**Prevelle Silk** and **Juvéderm XC**) are great for lips and mild smile lines; heavier ones (**Perlane** and **Juvéderm XC Plus**) are used to fill deep folds and accentuate cheekbones. **Belotero** is excellent for fine lines, especially around eyes and lips. These fillers are made from hyaluronic acid, a natural component of skin. The great thing about these fillers is that if the patient doesn't like the result, they can be dissolved with a simple injection. **Radiesse** is an entirely different type of filler; while in experienced hands it can be very good for deep folds, it does not dissolve for at least a year and has the potential for serious side effects.

FIFTY-THREE

Fillers Don't Last as Long on Happy People

Seriously, people who smile and laugh a lot use facial muscles that break down fillers more quickly—not that people should let that stop them from enjoying life. Even those who never crack a smile will find that lip fillers don't last as long as those in creases and cheekbones, because the only time lips are not in motion is when people are silent or asleep.

FIFTY-FOUR

Exercise Your Body, Not Your Face

Facial exercises are great—if you want more wrinkles. All those gizmos and facial exercise routines are nothing but scams. The more the face moves, the deeper the creases and wrinkles. Don't believe me? Look at somebody who has facial paralysis on just one side—the paralyzed side is always much smoother than the other side. That's the concept behind **Botox,** which paralyzes the muscle temporarily, making facial lines disappear.

FIFTY-FIVE

With Botox, Less Is More

Botox has an undeserved bad reputation for creating blank, expressionless faces because some doctors don't know how to use it properly. Before I inject Botox, I observe my patients carefully to see how they use their facial muscles. I don't like the unnatural, Stepford wife look myself. Some of my patients are models who ask for (and get) an absolutely smooth forehead, but that is not my signature look. I prefer the Botox "lite" approach that softens lines and creases but still allows expression; after all, the actors and newscasters who come to me want to be able to show emotion on camera. What I give them is such a soft, natural look that their viewers don't realize it is the result of Botox treatments. Botox alternatives are turning up on the market. **Dysport** and **Xeomin**, for example, are increasingly used and are just as effective.

Be very choosy about who is giving you Botox injections, because in inexperienced hands the results can be facial paralysis and slurred speech for several months. And always steer clear of Botox that seems suspiciously cheap, because it may be counterfeit or diluted. Either way, you are putting yourself at risk.

FIFTY-SIX

A Fuller Face Looks Younger

As we age, our faces lose bone and subcutaneous fat. The result is a thinner face that looks older. This is particularly true of people who keep themselves very lean. The remedy is volumizing the face, which can be done in two ways: with collagen stimulators like **Sculptra,** which take several treatments and months to see results, or with fillers where the results are instantaneous. Many of my patients like getting both: Sculptra for the long-term benefit, since the results can last two years, and fillers in the meantime. Fuller temples, cheeks, and jawline can make a huge difference, and increased collagen production means noticeably firmer skin.

FIFTY-SEVEN

Age Spots and Liver Spots Are Just Sun Spots

Those brown spots, which can really make people look old, can be prevented with regular use of sunscreen. If you already have them, they are easily treated with the **MedLite** or **Accutip** lasers, which take just seconds to zap each spot. There will be a scab for five to ten days, but when it falls off, your skin will have returned to its normal color. Very dark spots may require more than one treatment.

FIFTY-EIGHT

Laser Treatments Can Remove Many Signs of Sun Damage

People who sunbathe enthusiastically show damage everywhere. Splotched skin on their chests, brown spots on their arms and face—it's impossible to hide the ravages of the sun. But there is treatment available: The **LimeLight** and **Fraxel** lasers can go a long way toward repairing skin color. Many of my patients have it done all over their bodies, removing every trace of skin discoloration. Don't take this as a license to get tanned, though. Quite apart from the risk of skin cancer, sun damage can be very expensive to treat. A bottle of sunscreen costs less than $20, while treatment with a laser can run you several thousand dollars. Think about that.

FIFTY-NINE

Melasma Doesn't Have to Be Permanent

The hormones of pregnancy or birth control pills can lead to brown blotches on the face that do not go away after the baby is born or use of the pill is discontinued. Some people develop blotchy skin without the pill or the baby. The good news is that there are effective treatment options. The **Fraxel Re:Store Dual Wavelength** laser requires two or three treatments, but is highly effective. Some nonprescription creams do the job, too, especially when they're paired with retinoid creams, glycolic acid, or microdermabrasion. My favorites are **Neocutis Perle, Lumixyl,** and **Elure,** which are effective yet gentle on the skin. That is an important consideration: Melasma has to be handled very carefully, because overly aggressive treatment can make it worse. **Porcelana,** a 2% hydroquinone cream, is inexpensive and widely available, but not everybody tolerates hydroquinone. **Tri-Luma,** a prescription-only product, contains a higher percentage of hydroquinone. While it certainly lightens discolorations, it can also irritate sensitive skin.

Once the brown of melasma has faded, you must be hyper-vigilant about sun protection, or it will come back. And, I'm afraid, another pregnancy will almost always bring it back, too. The bottom line is that melasma is usually a recurring, albeit treatable, condition.

SIXTY

Treat Stretch Marks Early

Stretch marks aren't just for pregnant women. Anybody can get them, from men who lift weights to teenagers going through a dramatic growth spurt, because stretch marks are simple breaks in the elastic fibers of the skin. The bad news is that there is little you can do to prevent them; the good news is that you can do a lot to treat them. While no treatment will ever eliminate them completely, in many cases they can be made almost imperceptible, although darker skin is much harder to treat. If the stretch marks are red, it is essential to use sunscreen to protect the skin from further damage. If they are lasered in this early stage, the results will be even better. Once they fade to white, they can still be treated with lasers or with prescription tretinoin cream. Over-the-counter retinol creams work, but not to the same extent. Since tretinoin and retinol creams tend to dry out the skin, it is important to use a good moisturizer. Remember, use tretinoin and retinol creams only at night, never during the day.

SIXTY-ONE

Freeze Fat, Don't Suction It

L iposuction used to be the only alternative for people who wanted to remove or sculpt fat, even though it can be painful, has a fairly long and uncomfortable recovery period, and comes with serious potential side effects. But now we have **CoolSculpting, Liposonix,** and **truSculpt,** three revolutionary technologies. CoolSculpting freezes fat cells, Liposonix uses targeted ultrasound, and truSculpt is a radio frequency technology, but the end result for all three is the same: fat is gradually and painlessly broken down and metabolized, just as it would if you went on a diet. There are no needles or incisions. A month after the procedure, patients start noticing that their clothes fit more loosely; after four months, the results are comparable to liposuction.

CoolSculpting works best on large areas, such as substantial belly rolls or love handles; Liposonix and truSculpt treat small areas at a time, so they're best used to contour or sculpt the body, especially after a preliminary CoolSculpting treatment.

CoolSculpting is painless, and many people watch a movie or take a nap during treatment. Liposonix can be quite painful and uncomfortable, so ask for prescription painkillers and take them one hour before the procedure; truSculpt doesn't really hurt much, but the skin can get quite hot. Liposonix can be used on thighs and buttocks, truSculpt can be used anywhere beneath the neck, and CoolSculpting is currently limited to belly, love handles, and back fat.

In most cases, side effects of CoolSculpting and Liposonix are limited to a slight reddening and bruising, and occasionally mild muscle soreness; with truSculpt, side effects are rare. I tell my patients to avoid aspirin, alcohol, vitamin E and fish oil for a week before the procedure to minimize bruising.

CoolSculpting, Liposonix, and truSculpt will never replace the need to go to the gym or to keep to a healthy diet, but if you have unsightly bulges that bother you or want your waistline back, they are the safest, most effective way to go.

SIXTY-TWO

Tighten Before You Cut

As a doctor, I am more aware than most of the risks of going under anesthesia. That's why I am so delighted with the revolution in cosmetic dermatology, because it means that patients who want to improve their appearance can do so in a far safer way than surgery. One of the greatest advances is the use of sound waves and radio frequency to tighten the skin by stimulating collagen production instead of going for the traditional, under-the-knife face-lift. Some dermatologists have had good results with **Ulthera,** which uses focused ultrasound. In my practice we use **Thermage CPT** (which is not the same as plain **Thermage**), and I am here to say that it gives fabulous results. Unlike a face-lift, Thermage CPT does not cause swelling, bruising, or redness. Patients have their treatments as they chat about the dinner and play they are going to that evening. They usually see a difference almost immediately, but the remarkable part is that the skin continues to grow tighter and firmer for six months. The radio frequency stimulates collagen production. The change is gradual but noticeable, and never too tight or unnatural, which a face-lift can be.

Thermage CPT uses radio frequency and can be done anywhere on the body or face. The eye area usually shows the most dramatic results, because the skin is thinner and reacts faster. But Thermage CPT also has impressive results on sagging bellies and underarms. On bellies, the results after six months are comparable to surgical belly lifts. Thermage CPT can get rid of those drooping jowls and wrinkled knees, too. My middle-aged patients are thrilled to be able to wear short skirts again.

People always ask me if Thermage will get rid of cellulite. The answer is no, but because it will make the skin tighter and firmer, cellulite lumps will be less noticeable.

Some of those over-forty actresses who look astonishingly slim and taut have had Thermage done all over their bodies. Generally speaking, the firming effect lasts up to three years, but models and actresses sometimes get it every six months to maintain collagen production at its peak. I have to add that Thermage CPT is the most popular procedure in my office. Even I am stunned by the number of people who come to me wanting Thermage after seeing how it transformed a sister or a friend.

SIXTY-THREE

Laser Hair Removal Works

If Done Correctly

Laser hair removal can be tricky and you really need to be in experienced hands using the right equipment. If you have had two or three treatments without any significant reduction of hair, go elsewhere. In the wrong hands a laser can permanently damage your skin, so be very choosy.

The thing about laser hair removal is that it doesn't work for everybody. I always think of it as the brunettes' revenge, because blond or gray hair doesn't have enough pigment for the laser to work. For the treatment to be fully effective, the area has to be done every four to six weeks for about five months, because that way you are always zapping hair in the growth stage, which is when the laser works best. Lasers do a good job of removing hair from almost everywhere except the eyebrows, which are impossible to shape with a laser and should be treated with electrolysis.

SIXTY-FOUR

Alcohol and Razors Do Mix

Some people are just prone to red shaving bumps, especially if they have sensitive skin. An ultra-clean razor is essential. No matter what part of the body is to be shaved, always wait until after the shower, when hair is hydrated and softer. Before you step into the shower, place the razor in rubbing alcohol, so by the time you're ready the razor is disinfected. Use a shaving brush, which helps lift the hair off the skin, and a shaving gel instead of a cream. Don't shave against the direction of the hair, and do not go over the area more than once. If you get pimples, you will need a prescription antibiotic cream. In my practice, we have excellent results mixing a prescription antibiotic foam with shaving gel.

If you get a bikini wax, it's a good idea to apply an over-the-counter antibiotic or hydrocortisone cream immediately afterward. Wait a day or two before applying a self-tanner.

SIXTY-FIVE

Think Before You Ink

Every week I have patients come in for tattoo removals, which makes me wonder why people get them in the first place. Something people should know: A dermatologist can usually remove the tattoo with a laser, but there are several issues. First, it can take eight to ten treatments, so it is not cheap. Second, some colors are easier to remove than others: Black ink is easy to erase, but white and pale colors are almost impossible. Third, permanent makeup often cannot be removed and is a really stupid idea anyway. Permanent eyeliner cannot be treated because the laser would come dangerously close to the eye. Tattooed eyebrows are there forever because using a laser would destroy the hair follicles. And one more reason to avoid permanent makeup: It starts blurring with time, which means smudged lips and bleary-looking eyes.

That said, we do perform medical tattoos in my office. Women who have had breast reconstruction after mastectomies can get realistic-looking nipples tattooed. This is one area where a little blurring with time does not make much difference.

SIXTY-SIX

Clean Earrings Every Time You Put Them In

Earring posts—the part that goes through the lobe—can carry millions of bacteria. Always wipe them with alcohol before inserting, particularly if you are trying them on in the store. If you haven't followed this advice and you have an infection, dab some antibiotic ointment on the post, slip it in so the ointment penetrates all the way through, then remove the earring—and keep it removed until the infection clears up.

Many people are allergic to nickel, which means they have to use earrings with posts made of surgical stainless steel, titanium, gold, or platinum. While we're on the subject, I truly recommend that any piercing be done at a doctor's office to avoid the risk of infection and serious scarring.

For the middle-aged who love their earrings but hate

the way their aging earlobes have sagged, earlobes can be rejuvenated—I kid you not. Fillers can be used to plump and shorten lobes in a ten-minute office visit. As for torn lobes, most doctors can sew them up.

RULE #

SIXTY-SEVEN

For Hair Loss, Go

to a Doctor

There are so many medical reasons for hair loss (thyroid problems, anemia, lupus, to name a few), that the first thing anybody losing hair should do is get a complete medical checkup. If no medical issues are found, don't give up—there are some effective remedies available now. **Propecia** is a daily prescription pill that works well for men, although it has not been approved for women. However, some men have reported a serious side effect: temporary or permanent impotence. Before starting Propecia, make sure to discuss this with your doctor. **Minoxidil** works well on both sexes. (Note: Minoxidil should never be used by pregnant women or women who are breastfeeding.) While the commercial women's **Minoxidil** solution is only 2 percent, I have found that a 5 percent solution or foam, which is marketed only for men, works well on women. Women should use it only once a day, preferably at night. Be aware that some women report that this stronger concentration causes the growth of facial hair. One way to avoid this is to wash hands very, very carefully after applying minoxidil, so that no trace remains to be carried to the face. And be careful when applying it so that it does not drip down the face.

There is a good possibility that **Latisse,** which is so remarkable at growing eyelashes and eyebrows, may work on scalp hair, although probably in a stronger concentration. It's currently being studied for hair loss, but the manufacturer has yet to announce any definitive results.

Low-energy laser stimulation of the scalp, in at-home and in-office versions, seems to give mixed or at least unspectacular results.

RULE #

SIXTY-EIGHT

Chicken Skin Doesn't Belong on Humans

T hose tiny bumps (keratosis pilaris) some people have on their arms and legs are actually hereditary, but that doesn't mean they can't be treated. They cannot be scrubbed off, but gentle exfoliation does help, because it allows the skin to absorb treatments better. Look in the anti-acne section for products with salicylic acid, such as **Paula's Choice Exfoliating 2% Gel. AmLactin Body Moisturizing Lotion** with lactic acid, also works. If the bumps are red, you may need a little over-the-counter hydrocortisone cream. For really bad cases, ask for prescription **Kerafoam** or **Uramaxin,** which can really smooth the skin.

SIXTY-NINE

Take Biotin for Cracked, Brittle Nails

Far more effective than those "nail-strengthening" polishes is a daily dose of **biotin** (vitamin B-7), which can be purchased at any drugstore. Most recent studies recommend 2.5 milligrams a day. Interestingly, there is also some evidence that taking biotin regularly makes hair thicker and healthier, so it's a win-win situation. Anybody who has brittle or crumbling nails should ask their doctor about **Genadur,** a new prescription product. It's best applied like a polish on toenails and fingernails at night because it should not be washed off for several hours. A good over-the-counter alternative is **Barielle Nail Rebuilding Protein.** The best nail file I've found for fragile nails is the **Sassella Crystal Glass File.** Two very good files for all types of nails are the **Tweezerman Diamond** and the **OPI Crystal.**

While we're on the subject of nails: Avoid the UV heating lamps used in salons to speed the drying nail polish, because those UV rays age your hands. Let your nail polish dry naturally instead. And stay away from nail gels; more and more salons are offering them, but there are increasing reports of serious side effects, including neurological damage. They're so hard to get off that nails can be damaged easily in the process.

I am not a huge fan of nail extensions, and that is putting it mildly. People don't realize that the space between the fake nail and the real nail is the ideal environment for bacteria and fungi to grow. Sooner or later, people who use nail extensions are going to get an infection—and these infections are really nasty-looking and hard to treat. So if you like long nails, take biotin and grow your own instead.

SEVENTY

Don't Let Your Hands Show Your Age

People often don't realize that hands give away their age in an instant. It makes no sense to spend money to get a youthful, unlined face if your hands don't match. Ropy veins can be eliminated with an injection in a five-minute procedure. But you must always leave one vein untreated for future IV access; I say this as a doctor who worked in an emergency room. Those liver spots can be zapped with a laser, instantly erasing years; Skin lightening creams do not work on dark liver spots. The skin can be tightened with **Thermage CPT,** and finally a filler like **Radiesse** can plump up the hands and last an entire year. Honestly, a dermatologist can make a fifty-year-old hand look twenty-five again.

SEVENTY-ONE

Don't Let Them See You Sweat—Use Botox

No matter how fastidious people are about personal hygiene, some just seem to sweat a lot more. The result is big, wet rings under the arms that make people look nervous and ruin clothes. Until recently, the only remedies for excessive sweating were over-the-counter and prescription antiperspirants, which are not only drying and irritating, but not all that effective. **Botox** injections in the armpits, on the other hand, stop sweating there completely for a good six to seven months. Botox is not a cure, since it has to be done a couple of times a year, but it can eliminate what is a great source of embarrassment for some people.

Now, I do not recommend Botox shots for excessively sweaty hands and feet, because there is a serious risk of weakening muscles. Instead, buy or rent an iontophoresis machine, which uses water and electric current to decrease sweating. It sounds rather bizarre, but it actually works surprisingly well, so much so that some insurance companies cover the purchase of the equipment. A new procedure, **Miradry,** uses microwaves to zap sweat glands and drastically reduce sweat production. Although not yet widely available, the results appear to be encouraging.

By the way, antiperspirants are more effective when applied in the evening.

SEVENTY-TWO

Don't Scratch that Bug Bite

live in the most urban city in the world, and yet every week people come in to see me with bites from every insect imaginable, from bedbugs to spiders. No matter where you live, at some point you are going to be bitten. For the inevitable bites, here are a few tips. First, put an ice cube on the bite to relieve the itch instantly and to bring down the swelling. Then use alcohol and an over-the-counter cortisone cream. Milk and water compresses also work. If it's really bad, take an over-the-counter Benadryl pill (never use an antihistamine spray; it can cause an allergic reaction). And if you have any wheezing or trouble breathing, get yourself to an emergency room immediately—you may be having an anaphylactic reaction.

It's really important to treat the itch because scratching can scar the skin and can easily lead to serious staph infections.

SEVENTY-THREE

Keep All Cuts and Scratches Moist for Better Healing

Even minor abrasions can leave scars. To speed healing and minimize scarring, always clean the area with alcohol, apply **Aquaphor Healing Ointment** or a topical antibiotic ointment (a cream is not as effective) such as **Bacitracin,** and cover with a **Band-Aid.** If the cut or abrasion is on the face, use **DuoDerm Extra-Thin Dressing,** an innovative product that promotes healing. Never clean wounds with hydrogen peroxide because it slows healing.

SEVENTY-FOUR

Surgical Scars Can Be Minimized

ny surgical scar, including those from cesarean sections, can be reduced with the use of a special silicone bandage. I always tell my patients that if they have any surgeries planned, they should get bandages even before they go to the hospital. People who have a tendency to form keloids should definitely invest in them. You have to wait until the stitches are out, but I do think that the sooner you start using them, the better the results. Silicone bandages also work on old scars. The brand I recommend is **Mepiform,** but there are other good, less expensive alternatives, such as **ScarAway Silicone Sheets.**

If the scarring is severe, there are other options. Laser treatments can flatten raised scars and blend color into surrounding skin. Steroid injections and steroid-impregnated strips can also flatten. When all else fails, the scar can be cut out and the new scar minimized from the beginning with steroids and silicone bandages. It is very important to protect recent scars from the sun; use a physical sunscreen, preferably one with zinc oxide.

SEVENTY-FIVE

Drink Green Tea—Lots of It

t seems that every week scientists discover new benefits from drinking green tea. We now know that it aids weight loss by boosting metabolism, for example, but there is increasing evidence that green tea also has very specific effects on the skin. It is full of polyphenols, antioxidants that appear to prevent skin cancer and protect against free radicals that age the skin. White tea has even more polyphenols, but it also costs more and some find it less flavorful. Green tea is a preventive, not a cure, so the key here is to start drinking it at an early age and to drink it every day. The ideal dose is four cups a day, but if peeing a lot doesn't appeal, green tea supplements work well, as long as they are standardized. The dose I recommend is 500 milligrams daily.

Three tips: First, adding lemon or lime to a cup of green tea increases its effectiveness. Second, green tea is an anti-inflammatory, so an application of green tea (let it cool first, obviously) soothes irritated skin or a mild sunburn. Third, bottled green tea may taste good, but it does not have the same benefits as freshly brewed tea.

I have become such a fan of green tea that I not only drink several cups a day, I also offer it to patients in my practice. One thing I have learned, though: Don't drink green tea (or anything with caffeine) after 5 P.M. if you want a good night's sleep. That goes for chocolate, too, since it contains caffeine.

RULE #

SEVENTY-SIX

Eat Right to Look Good

People need to eat protein for healthy skin and hair, but this does not mean huge quantities of ribs and steak. Eating small amounts of lean protein like fish, egg white omelets, or turkey will improve skin, hair, and nails without increasing weight. Skin needs healthy fats, too, like those found in fish, extra-virgin olive oil, and nuts. I also recommend that everybody take a 1,000 milligram omega-3 supplement daily.

Eat lots of fruit and vegetables. Pick the more colorful varieties, as they are usually more beneficial. For example, a pink grapefruit has fifty times more vitamin A than white grapefruit. Fresh or frozen berries are also an excellent choice, especially blueberries. Resist the temptation to have them with milk as it blocks the absorption of the antioxidants.

If you have acne, keep in mind that consuming dairy

products and sugar can make it worse. If you do eliminate dairy, be sure to take calcium supplements.

Remember, you can use the most expensive products in the world and have the best dermatologist, but if you are not eating correctly, your skin will show it.

SEVENTY-SEVEN

Beauty Sleep Is No Myth

When people don't get enough sleep, their cortisol levels rise, causing havoc throughout the body. This stress is reflected in skin, which is why people who toss and turn look so haggard in the morning. So if you want to look good, do everything you can to get a good night's sleep. And perhaps invest in 100 percent silk pillowcases—many people report that they wake up with fewer sleep wrinkles when they use them.

Acknowledgments

I want to thank my family for their love and support: my mother, Reva Jaliman; my brother, Michael Jaliman; my daughter, Alexa; and my love, Stephen Wang.

I wish to give thanks to my creative writing teacher, Alan Ziegler, who saw promise in me and encouraged me to write, and my friend M. E. Elliott, whose useful critiques helped shape this book.

This book could never have been finished without the help of my staff, including Agnes, Ana, Faye, Karla, Lissette, Weronika, and their invaluable assistance; I thank them all.

Every day I learn something new from my patients; this book could never have been written without them.

Resource Section

PRODUCTS

All Free and Clear: www.all-laundry.com

AmLactin: www.amlactin.com

Aquaphor: www.aquaphorhealing.com

Atopiclair: www.atopiclair.com

Aveeno: www.aveeno.com

Avene: www.aveneusa.com

Bacitracin: www.ferapharma.com

Badger Balm: www.badgerbalm.com

Band Aid: www.bandaid.com

CeraVe: www.cerave.com

Cetaphil: www.cetaphil.com

Cheer Free: www.cheer.com

Clarins: www.clarins.com

Clarisonic: www.clarisonic.com

Clinique: www.clinique.com

Colorescience: www.colorescience.com

DDF Revolve: www.ddfskincare.com

Diamancel: www.diamancel.com

Dr. Scholl's: www.drscholls.com

Duoderm: www.convatec.com

Elta: www.eltamd.com

Epiceram: www.epiceram.com

Essie: www.essie.com

Eucerin: www.eucerin.com

Genadur: www.meimetriks.com

Hampton Sun: www.hamptonsuncare.com

Heliocare: www.heliocare.com

Hylatopic Foam: www.onsetdermatologics.com

Jergens: www.jergens.com

Josie Maran Cosmetics: www.josiemaron.com

Journee: www.neocutis.com

Kerofoam: www.onsetdermatologics.com

Kiehl's: www.kiehls.com

Lancome: www.lancome-usa.com

La Roche Posay: www.laroche-posav.us

Lashdip: www.lashdip.com

Latisse: www.latisse.com

Lorac: www.loraccosmetics.com

L'Oreal: www.loreal.com

Lumixyl: www.lumixyl.net

Mepiform: www.directmedicalinc.com

Mimyx: www.stiefel.com

Minoxidil: www.minoxidil.com

Murad: www.murad.com

Mustela: www.mustelausa.com

NeoCutis (Perle): www.neocutis.com

Neova: www.photomedex.com

Neutrogena: www.neutrogena.com

Oilatum: www.stiefel.com

Olay: www.olay.com

Ole Henriksen: www.olehenriksen.com

Paula's Choice: www.paulaschoice.com

Peter Thomas Roth: www.peterthomasroth.com
Philosophy: www.philosophy.com
Physicians Formula: www.physiciansformula.com
Propecia: www.propecia.com
Pyratine XR: www.pyratineXR.com
Rapid Lash: www.rapidlash.com
Revitalash: www.revitalash.com
RoC: www.rocskincare.com
Roux: www.sallybeauty.com
ScarAway: www.myscaraway.com
Shiseido: www.shiseido.com
Skinceuticals: www.skinceuticals.com
Skin Medica: www.skinmedica.com
Stila: www.stilacosmetics.com
Stridex: www.stridex.com
St.Tropez: www.sttropeztan.com
Tide Free: www.tide.com
Triluma: www.triluma.com
Trish McEvoy: www.trishmcevoy.com
Tweezerman: www.tweezerman.com
Uramaxin: www.medimetriks.com
Vanicream: www.psico.com
Vaseline: www.vaseline.com
Zo Skin Health: www.zoskinhealth.com

INJECTABLES (Facial Fillers/Stimulants/Neurotoxins)
Facial fillers from lightest to heaviest
Prevelle: www.prevelle.com
Juvederm: www.juvederm.com
Restylane: www.restylaneusa.com
Perlane: www.perlanecosmetic.com
Radiesse: www.radiesse.com

Collagen stimulant

Sculptra: www.sculptraaesthetic.com

Neurotoxins

Botox: www.botoxcosmetic.com

Dysport: www.dysportusa.com

Lasers and other in-office procedures

Acutip: www.cutera.com/

CoolGlide: www.cutera.com/

CoolSculpting by Zeltiq: www.coolsculpting.com

Fraxel: www.fraxel.com

LimeLight: www.cutera.com/

MedLite: www.conbio.com/

Thermage CPT: www.thermage.com

Ulthera: www.ulthera.com

SUN-PROTECTIVE CLOTHING

More and more companies are selling sun-protective clothing. Below are links to a few and to Sunguard, a powder that can be used in laundry to add sun protection to clothes you already own.

Coolibar: www.coolibar.com

L.L. Bean: www.llbean.com

Mott 50: www.mott50.com

Solumbra: www.sunprecautions.com

Sunguard: www.sunguardsunprotection.com